Gluten-Fre Beginners

Create Your Gluten-Free Lifestyle for Vibrant Health, Wellness and Weight Loss (Mouth-Watering Recipes Included)

By Kira Novac

ISBN: 978-1-80095-009-2

Table of Contents

Introduction

It seems as though a new fad diet hits the newsstands every couple of weeks. Some celebrity is always coming out with a new secret to staying skinny and nutritionists debate the merits of the most recent cleanse or detox. The gluten-free diet is by no means new, but it has become newly popularized over the last decade or so. Many people switch to this diet under the misguided impression that it will help them to magically lose weight while others simply make the switch to follow the latest trend. Before you switch to the popular gluten-free diet, you should take a moment to learn the basics about this diet including its benefits, risks, and what exactly the diet entails.

My name is Kira and I am a 35-year-old mother of one. A few years ago, my son was diagnosed with celiac (also called celiac sprue) disease and, while the diagnosis came as a bit of a shock, I am glad to finally have an answer to my son's health problems. When my son was diagnosed I made the decision to not only provide him with the gluten-free diet he needed, but to create a healthy lifestyle for myself and my entire family. We have never really been a fast food family, but I am ashamed to admit that frozen dinners and take-out appeared on our weekly menu more often than they should have. Now, however, I am committed to cooking for my family several times a week and we have all made the switch to the gluten-free diet for the benefit of my son.

While this type of diet is not some magical weight loss pill, it does have a number of benefits even for people without celiac disease and those without gluten sensitivities. Many people suffer from a condition called gluten intolerance and they do not even realize it - switching to the gluten-free diet can completely transform their lives. Removing gluten from your diet can help to improve and regulate your digestion and it may provide relief from mood disorders and problems with concentration. Each person reacts to the gluten-free diet differently, but I am a firm believer that it can be a useful tool if you want to improve your health and transform your life.

Committing to the gluten-free diet is not easy and it isn't a decision you should take lightly. If you are thinking about making the switch it is my hope that this book will provide you with the information you need in order to make a well-informed decision. If you do decide that the gluten-free diet is right for you, you will find a collection of delicious recipes in this book that I have created for my family and am now sharing with you. Try a few recipes to see how you like them and you might be surprised just how easy it is to switch to the gluten-free diet.

If you are ready to learn more about this diet and how it can benefit you, turn the page and keep reading!

About the Gluten-Free Diet

Before you decide whether the gluten-free diet is the right choice for you, you need to learn everything you can about the diet. The gluten-free diet is more than just another fad diet – it is intended to be a lifestyle choice and one that many people follow out of medical necessity. The gluten-free diet is quite simple – it is a diet that is completely free from gluten-containing foods. In order to understand the gluten-free diet, you first need to understand what gluten is and where it comes from.

What is Gluten?

Gluten is a type of protein composite and it is commonly found in certain grains including wheat, barley, rye, and triticale (a hybrid form of wheat). Gluten is a composite made up of two storage proteins – glutenin and gliadin – which are joined with a starch. This protein composite is found in the endosperm of several grass-like grains and it is what gives bread dough its elasticity, rise, and chewy texture. Gluten can be found in a wide variety of different foods because it is found in wheat flour and it is commonly used to thicken liquid foods like soups and sauces.

4

On its own, gluten is not necessarily bad – it is primarily bad for people who have celiac disease or other gluten-related conditions like allergies, intolerance, or sensitivity. It is estimated that about 1 in 133 people have celiac disease, an autoimmune disease exacerbated by the consumption of gluten, and that millions of people suffer from some kind of gluten-related intolerance or sensitivity. It is also estimated that about 99% of people who suffer from problems related to gluten aren't even aware of it because the symptoms of gluten intolerance or sensitivity overlap with the symptoms of many other diseases.

Why is Gluten Bad?

Again, gluten is not necessarily bad, but it can cause problems for those people who suffer from certain conditions including celiac disease and gluten intolerance or sensitivity. The symptoms of celiac disease vary greatly from one person to another which makes it very difficult to diagnose. In some individuals with celiac disease gluten causes digestive issues like diarrhea, gas, or bloating. In others, however, it causes fatigue, brain fog, weight loss, anxiety, depression, as well as many other mental/behavioral symptoms.

Celiac disease is an autoimmune condition, though many people mistakenly believe it is a type of allergy. When a person with celiac disease consumes gluten, their body regards the gluten protein as a foreign invader and produces an immune response. In addition to targeting the gluten, however, the immune cells end up attacking healthy cells in the small intestine as well. As a result, the villi lining the small intestine become damaged and it may result in the malabsorption of nutrients – this is likely the cause of certain celiac disease-related symptoms like chronic fatigue.

Gluten intolerance is a completely different condition. While individuals with celiac disease experience an immune response when they consume gluten, individuals with gluten intolerance typically experience gastrointestinal symptoms like diarrhea, bloating, gas, and abdominal pain. Celiac disease is similar to an extreme form of gluten intolerance, but it is possible to have a gluten intolerance without having celiac disease. The only treatment for either condition is to follow a gluten-free diet.

In individuals with celiac disease or gluten intolerance/sensitivity, consuming gluten can result in several serious problems including the following:

- Gut inflammation

- Autoimmune response

- Premature cell death and oxidation

- Leaky gut syndrome

- Bacterial overgrowth in the intestinal tract

- Vitamin D deficiency

For these reasons, it is very important that individuals diagnosed with celiac disease, gluten intolerance, and/or gluten sensitivity completely remove gluten from their diets. This is the only proven treatment that will result in relief from symptoms.

Gluten-Containing Foods

Switching to the gluten-free diet can be tricky because gluten is found in so many foods. Not only is it found in baked goods made from wheat and other gluten-containing grains, but it is also commonly found in other foods like fried foods, Asian-style sauces, soups, beer, snack foods, cereals, and more. Fortunately, most food labels for commercially-produced foods carry an allergy statement which will tell you if the product contains wheat. There are some ingredients, however, in which gluten can be hiding that you may not suspect.

For example, anything with "malt" in the ingredients is typically made from barley and is therefore not gluten-free. Breaded meats, commercial sauces, thickened soups, and most beer is also not gluten-free. Even oats, which are technically gluten-free, can be contaminated by coming into contact with wheat grains during processing. <u>Below you will find a list of common foods that typically contain gluten</u>:

- Sauces
- Soy sauce
- Teriyaki sauce
- Licorice
- Imitation crab meat

- Self-basting turkey
- Spelt
- Wheat
- Kamut
- Triticale

- Durum
- Einkorn
- Farina
- Semolina
- Cake flour
- Matzo

- Couscous
- Barley
- Rye
- Bread
- Pastries
- Breakfast cereal
- Cakes and pies
- Bagels and biscuits
- Muffins
- Pizza dough

- Pumpernickel
- Malt beverages
- Malt syrup
- Malt flavoring
- Malt powder
- Malt vinegar
- Beer
- Blue cheese
- Processed cheese

- Seasoning mixes
- Soups
- Snack mixes
- Non-dairy creamer
- Sausages
- Hot dogs
- Stuffing mixes
- Pretzels
- Snack bars

This list is not exhaustive, but it will give you a good idea what type of foods and products typically contain gluten.

Gluten-Free Foods

Looking at the list from the last section, you might be wondering what foods are left. Though it is true that gluten is found in a wide variety of different foods, most unprocessed foods are naturally gluten-free. This includes things like fresh fruits, vegetables, herbs, nuts, seeds, eggs, meats, and oils. Most dairy products aside from malted milk, blue cheese, and certain flavors of yogurt and ice cream are also free from gluten-containing ingredients.

As an alternative to gluten-containing flours like all-purpose flour and wheat flour there are many flours made from nuts or non-gluten-containing grains that you can use to make gluten-free versions of your favorite recipes. <u>Below you will find a list of gluten-free flours and baking substitutes</u>:

- Amaranth flour
- Arrowroot powder
- Almond flour
- Baking powder
- Baking soda
- Buckwheat flour
- Chestnut flour
- Chia seed flour
- Coconut flour
- Corn flour
- Cornstarch
- Garbanzo bean flour
- Ground flaxseed
- Hazelnut flour
- Mesquite flour
- Millet flour
- Oat flour
- Potato flour
- Potato starch
- Soy flour
- Tapioca flour
- Tapioca starch
- Quinoa flour
- Rice flour
- Sorghum flour
- Teff flour
- Xanthan gum

In fact, you can make your own gluten-free flour blends to use in your favorite recipes. To make a gluten-free flour blend, simply combine equal parts of two different gluten-free flours with an equal portion of a gluten-free starch. Most gluten-free flours and starches will work well with this ratio except for almond flour and potato flour.

Avoiding Cross-Contamination

When you make the switch to the gluten-free diet you need to do more than just avoid gluten-containing ingredients – you also need to avoid cross-contamination. This is especially important for individuals with celiac disease because they may have a reaction to even the smallest amount of gluten. Cross-contamination happens when a food that is gluten-free comes into direct or indirect contact with a food or ingredient that contains gluten. This can happen during the manufacturing process for commercial foods or in your very own kitchen. If you do not plan on having your entire family make the switch to the gluten-free diet, you may need to keep two different containers of certain products like peanut butter, jams/jellies, and butter to make sure that cross-contamination isn't a problem.

When eating out on the gluten-free diet it is important that you let your server and the cook know about your dietary restrictions. Many recipes offer gluten-free items on their menus but you still need to be sure that they take precautions against cross-contamination. For example, your dish needs to be prepared with clean utensils in a pot or pan that hasn't come into contact with gluten-containing ingredients. Some restaurants even keep separate utensils and cookware for use in preparing gluten-free menu items.

While the gluten-free diet is rapidly gaining in popularity, many people still have a poor understanding of the diet. This being the case, you need to be very careful when you go out to eat. You may even want to call the restaurant ahead of time and speak to the manager to make sure that they can accommodate your dietary restrictions. Do not assume that everyone knows what celiac disease is, or even what gluten is, and do not hesitate to educate people when necessary to make sure that you do not become a victim of cross-contamination.

Risks Associated with the Gluten-Free Diet

As is true for any diet, switching to the gluten-free diet does come with certain risks. Individuals who follow gluten-free diets have been known to exhibit lower than normal levels of certain vitamins and minerals including iron, fiber, calcium, thiamin, niacin, riboflavin, and folate. Ask your doctor about supplements and always be sure to check with him before making any changes to your diet. Once you switch over to the gluten-free diet (especially if you have celiac disease or a gluten intolerance/sensitivity), your body may produce severe reactions if you accidentally ingest a little gluten. The longer you follow the gluten-free diet without deviation, the more severe your reaction will be in cases like this. Even if you do not experience physical symptoms after eating gluten, it could still be doing damage to your intestines.

Because the gluten-free diet has become more popular of late, gluten-free versions of many processed foods are becoming more widely available. Of course, these foods are often much more expensive than the regular version with some products costing double (or more) the price of the traditional version. Many people who switch to the gluten-free diet without doing their research (especially those who don't have a medical necessity for following the diet) do not realize that gluten-free versions of processed foods are still processed foods – they can still be high in calories, fat, and sugar. Just because something is gluten-free doesn't necessarily make it healthy. You still need to monitor your calorie intake on a gluten-free diet and make healthy food choices such as portion control.

If you suffer from celiac disease or have a gluten intolerance/sensitivity, switching to the gluten-free diet may not be choice – it could be a medical necessity. Even those who do not have a medical need to follow the diet can still benefit from removing gluten-from their diet, however. If you are considering switching to the gluten-free diet, take the information from this chapter to heart and talk to your doctor before making the switch. If you decide that the gluten-free diet is indeed the right choice for you, give some of the recipes in this book a try!

The Gluten-Free Diet for Weight Loss

Here comes another benefit of going gluten-free. If you do it the right way, you can lose weight. The mere fact of eliminating gluten products from your diet does not automatically guarantee weight loss, however, if you follow my recommendations, you will start losing weight naturally. Once and for all. Without feeling deprived or going hungry.

Personally, before going gluten-free, I tried many diets and programs. Nothing worked long-term. I got sick and tired of counting calories and finally, I accepted my extra pounds. OK, self-love and acceptance are important but what was worrying me was that I would get fatter and fatter and I had no energy. This is why I was really happy I switched to a gluten-free lifestyle. Read on to discover a few simple tricks to speed up your weight loss success while sticking to a gluten-free diet.

A gluten-free diet will assist you in losing weight. One way that it does this is obvious. All of the foods you will be eating are very healthy and natural. You will eliminate processed high-carb stuff (pasta, rice, cookies, bread) and switch to healthier alternatives. All you need to do is to:

- Add more vegetables into your diet (especially green vegetables as there are very alkalizing)

- Eliminate processed sugar (my snack and dessert recipes will help you satisfy your sweet tooth without feeling deprived)

- Try to stick to a Paleo gluten-free lifestyle as much as possible and eliminate cheese (you can have some cheese on a gluten-free diet, however if your weight loss is also your goal, I suggest you stick to a Paleo style plan that consists of lean protein, fish, nuts, seeds, plenty of fruits and vegetables). Some of the recipes from this book contain a bit of cheese for variety and since my main goal was to write a gluten-free diet guide that is easy to follow for beginners, I did not want to come up with the recipes that might be too restrictive or too hard to make a transition. The bottom line is- if you want to lose weight- reduce or eliminate cheese and dairy products. Organic eggs are fine.

- Drink plenty of fresh water, personally I recommend alkaline water (a simple pitcher with filters will do and it will also save you money in the long-run)

- Add more alkaline foods into your diet. All highly alkalizing foods are also gluten-free. Try to sneak in as many greens as you can. If you can stick to a gluten-free diet and enrich it with more alkaline foods, you will be losing weight naturally. Why?

Well, you will also be reducing the amount of acid in your body. The body stores fat to protect itself from an abundance of acid. It is a self-preservation method. This is part of the reason why people who exercise a lot and do fad diets cannot seem to lose those extra pounds. Their bodies are clinging to that fat to minimize the effects of all the acid in their systems.

Another benefit of a gluten-free alkaline lifestyle regarding weight loss is that alkaline systems have more oxygen in their cells. Oxygen is a very essential part of eliminating fat cells from the body. The more oxygen in your system, the more efficient your metabolism will be. So again- eat more raw, alkaline foods. These are natural gluten-free.

As you may have realized, gluten is acid-forming. Those who follow an alkaline diet, also try to avoid gluten for health reasons.

Simply by eliminating gluten from your diet and adding more natural, fresh foods, salads, fruits and veggies, you will have much more energy. This is what happened to me and, so I took this "new energy" with me to the gym. The effect was very fast and first time in my life I enjoyed working out.

So, to sum up- use my recipes as a staple. They will help you feel full and create a gluten-free lifestyle without feeling deprived. Additionally, try to add more alkaline foods into your diet. They will help your body regulate your pH so that you feel more energetic.

Let me just give you a list for quick reference:

Alkaline Fruits and Vegetables:

- Avocado
- Coconut
- Currants
- Grapefruit
- Lemon/Lime
- Tomato
- Alfalfa
- Barley Grass
- Beet
- Broccoli
- Cabbages
- Carrot
- Cauliflower
- Celery
- Cucumber
- Dandelions
- Eggplant
- Garlic
- Greens
- Kale
- Lettuces
- Onions
- Parsnips
- Peppers
- Pumpkin
- Radishes
- Rutabaga
- Sea weed
- Sprouts
- Tomato
- Watercress
- Wheat-Grass

Why you should back up your gluten-free lifestyle with fresher alkaline fruits and veggies?

The lymph fluids function most efficiently in an alkaline system. They remove acid waste. Acidic systems not only have a slower lymph flow causing acids to be stored; they can also cause acids to be reabsorbed through lymphatic ducts in your intestines that would normally be excreted

Also, please realize that during all your "gluten-years" you were putting way too many acidic foods in your body (all foods that contain gluten are acid-forming). By alkalizing your gluten-free diet, not only will you lose weight faster and in an all-natural way, but you will also reap off the following benefits:

- The liver's job is to get rid of acid toxins, but also to produce alkaline enzymes. By simply reducing your acid/gluten intake and adding more alkaline foods, you can internally boost your alkalinity thanks to your liver!

- Your pancreas thrives on alkalinity. Too much acid in your system throws off your pancreas. If you eat gluten-free, alkaline foods, your pancreas can regulate your blood sugars.

- Your kidneys also help to keep your body alkaline. When they are overwhelmed by an acidic, gluten-FULL diet they cannot do their job (and no one wants a kidney stone...)

Another huge benefit of a gluten-free lifestyle with an alkaline touch is detoxification. First, you're going to be cutting out foods that are constantly adding toxins to your system (gluten is very toxic). Secondly, you are going to be eating foods that allow your body to detox and rid itself of the acids that have built up in your system all this time. When we detoxify our bodies, our emotions, bodily functions and mental functions are able operate at their optimum levels.

This book is intended as a beginner's guide. However, I am now in the process of writing more advanced gluten-free guides, including: Paleo Gluten-Free, Alkaline Gluten-Free and even Vegan Gluten-Free. If you would like to be the first one to grab them for free, make sure you join my newsletter. As a special gift I will send you a free gluten-free recipe book full of delicious treats...

FREE EBOOK

Irresistible Gluten Free Desserts, Snacks & Treats

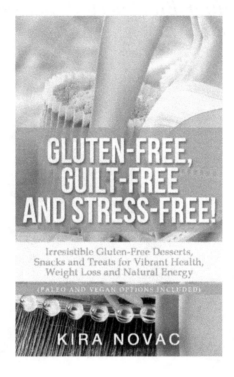

You can download your free recipe eBook at:

http://www.bit.ly/gluten-free-books

Now, let's jump into the recipes!

Breakfast Recipes

Almond-Flour Blueberry Pancakes
Servings: 4 to 5

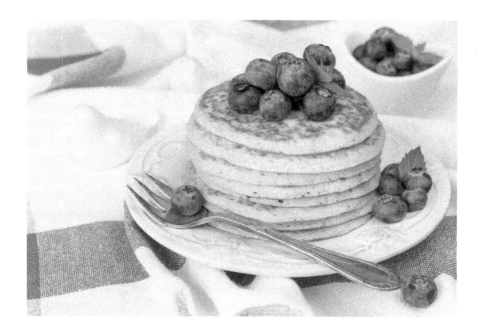

Ingredients:

- ¼ cup unsweetened almond milk
- 2 large eggs plus 2 whites, beaten
- 1 tablespoon unsalted butter, melted
- 1 tablespoon cane sugar
- ½ tablespoon vanilla extract

- ½ teaspoon distilled white vinegar
- 1 ½ cups almond flour
- ¾ teaspoon baking soda
- Pinch salt
- 1 to 1 ½ cups fresh blueberries

Instructions:

1. Preheat an electric griddle to high heat or a large nonstick skillet over the medium heat setting.
2. Combine the milk, eggs, and butter with the sugar, vanilla extract, and the white vinegar in a regular food processor.
3. Blend the mixture of wet ingredients until it is smooth and well combined.
4. Combine the remaining ingredients except for the fresh blueberries in a medium mixing bowl and stir them well.
5. Add the dry ingredients to the food processor and blend smooth.
6. Spoon the batter into the preheated griddle, using up to 3 tablespoons per pancake.
7. Sprinkle a few fresh blueberries into the wet batter for each pancake and cook the pancakes for 1 to 2 minutes until bubbles form in the surface of the batter.

8. Carefully flip the pancakes and cook for another minute or two until the underside is browned.

9. Transfer the pancakes to a plate to keep warm and repeat with the rest of the batter.

10. Serve the pancakes warm drizzled with maple syrup.

Cheesy Eggs in Avocado
Servings: 6

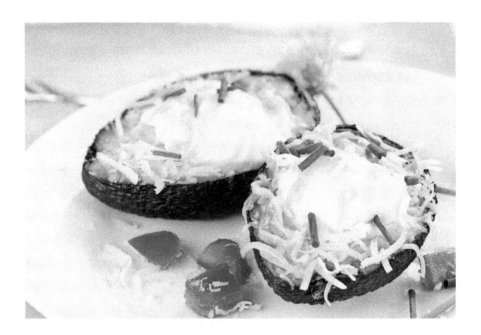

Ingredients:

- 3 ripe avocadoes
- 6 large eggs
- 1 cup shredded cheese (your choice)
- Salt and pepper to taste
- 3 tablespoons fresh chopped chives

Instructions:

1. Preheat your oven to a temperature of 425°F.
2. Carefully slice the fresh avocados into halves and then remove the pits.
3. Scoop out a tablespoon or two of flesh from the middle of each of the avocado halves then place them cut-side up in a baking dish.
4. Crack one egg into the depression in the center of each avocado then season the egg with the salt and pepper.
5. Sprinkle the cheese over the avocados and bake for 16 to 18 minutes until the eggs are cooked to the desired level.
6. Garnish with fresh chopped chives to serve.

Coconut-Flour Banana Muffins

Servings: 12

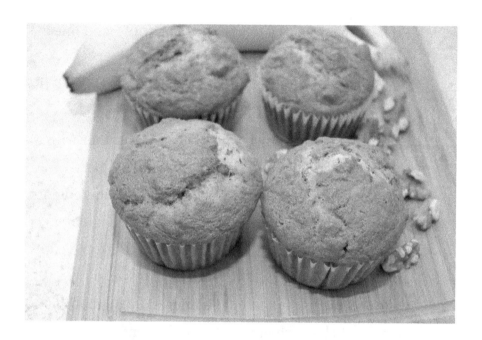

Ingredients:

- ½ cup sifted coconut flour
- ¾ teaspoon baking soda
- Pinch salt
- 5 large eggs, beaten well
- ¼ cup coconut oil
- 2 tablespoons of almond milk
- 1 ½ teaspoon almond extract

- 2 medium bananas, mashed

Instructions:

1. Preheat the oven to a temperature of 400°F and line a regular muffin pan with paper liners.
2. Combine the coconut flour and the baking soda with the salt in a mixing bowl then stir well.
3. In another mixing bowl, whisk the eggs together with the coconut oil, the milk and the almond extract.
4. Stir the wet ingredients into the bowl of dry ingredients until well combined then fold in the mashed banana.
5. Spoon the batter into the prepared pan, filling the cups about ¾ full.
6. Bake the muffins for 14 to 18 minutes until a toothpick comes out clean when inserted in the center of a muffin.
7. Cool the muffins for 5 minutes in the pan then turn out onto a wire rack and leave to cool completely.

Paleo Tomato Basil Omelet
Servings: 1

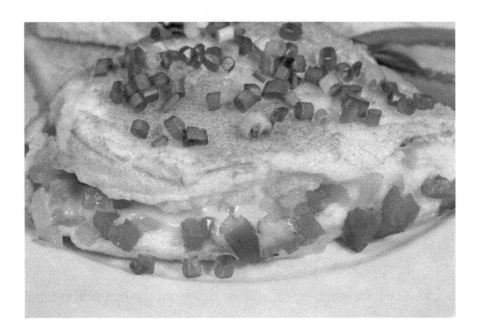

Ingredients:

- 2 teaspoons coconut oil
- 1 medium ripe tomato, chopped
- 2 to 3 tablespoons sweet onion, chopped
- Salt and pepper to taste
- 2 large eggs, whisked well
- 1 tablespoon fresh chopped chives
- 5 to 6 leaves fresh basil, chopped

Instructions:

1. Heat 1 teaspoon oil in a small nonstick skillet over medium-high heat.

2. Add the tomato and onion then season lightly with salt and pepper.

3. Cook for 1 to 2 minutes until the onion is translucent then spoon off into a small bowl.

4. Reheat the skillet using the remaining oil.

5. In a small bowl, beat the egg with the chives – pour the mixture of ingredients into the skillet and lightly season again with salt and pepper.

6. Let the egg cook for about 1 minute then swirl the pan to spread the uncooked egg.

7. Cook for another minute or two until the egg is almost set.

8. Spoon the cooked vegetables over half the omelet and sprinkle with basil.

9. Fold the empty half of the omelet over the fillings.

10. Cook for 1 minute or so more until the egg is set – slide onto a plate and serve hot.

Cheddar Broccoli Egg Cups
Servings: 3 to 4

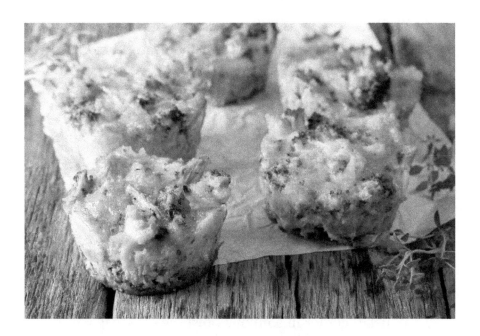

Ingredients:

- 4 cups broccoli florets, chopped
- 1 ½ teaspoons olive oil
- Salt and pepper to taste
- 6 large eggs plus 1 cup whites
- ¾ cup shredded cheddar cheese

Instructions:

1. Preheat your oven to a temperature of 350°F and grease the cups of a regular-sized muffin pan with your favorite cooking spray.
2. Fill a saucepan with about 1 inch of water then place a metal steamer insert in it.
3. Add the broccoli to the saucepan then cover it and bring the water to a boil – steam the broccoli for a few minutes until it is just tender.
4. Remove the broccoli and let cool slightly before chopping.
5. Toss the broccoli with the olive oil and season it with the salt and pepper.
6. Divide the broccoli mixture among the muffin cups.
7. Whisk together in a mixing bowl the eggs, egg whites and cheese – season the mixture with salt and pepper.
8. Fill the muffin cups the rest of the way with the blended egg and cheese mixture.
9. Bake for 18 to 20 minutes, or until the egg is completely set.

Double Chocolate Chip Waffles
Servings: 8 to 10

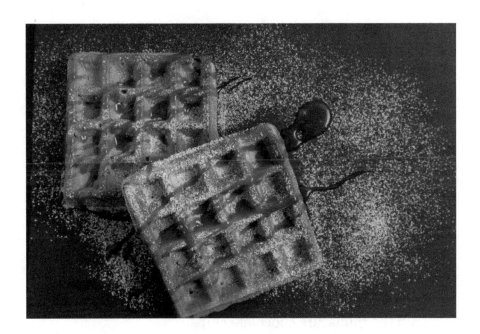

Ingredients:

- 2 cups gluten-free flour blend
- 6 tablespoons unsweetened cocoa powder
- 2 ½ tablespoon granulated sugar
- 1 ¾ teaspoons baking powder
- 1 teaspoon of xanthan gum
- ¼ teaspoon salt
- 2 cups unsweetened almond milk
- 6 tablespoons coconut oil, melted

- 2 large eggs, whisked well
- 1 ½ teaspoon vanilla extract
- ¾ cup miniature chocolate chips

Instructions:

1. Combine the gluten-free flour mix, cocoa powder, and sugar, with the xanthan gum, baking powder, and salt in a mixing bowl.
2. In a separate mixing bowl, beat together the almond milk and coconut oil with the eggs and the vanilla extract until smooth.
3. Whisk the wet ingredients into the bowl of dry ingredients until smooth and well combined then fold in the miniature chocolate chips.
4. Cover the bowl and let the batter rest at room temperature for 30 minutes.
5. Preheat your waffle iron according to the waffle maker's instructions.
6. Spoon the batter into the waffle iron, using the amount recommended in the instructions.
7. Close the waffle iron and cook according to the directions.
8. Remove the waffle to a plate to keep warm and repeat with the rest of the batter.

9. Serve the waffles warm drizzle with chocolate syrup or maple syrup.

Vegan Apple Cinnamon Muffins
Servings: 12

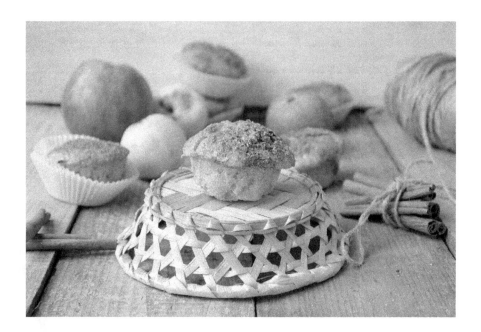

Ingredients:

- 1 ½ tablespoon flaxseed meal

- 2 ½ tablespoons warm water

- 3 teaspoons coconut oil

- 2 large ripe apples, diced

- 1 cup unsweetened coconut milk beverage

- ¾ cups unsweetened applesauce

- ½ cup coconut sugar

- 3 tablespoons vegetable oil

- ½ tablespoon vanilla extract
- 1 ½ cups gluten-free flour blend
- 1 ½ teaspoon ground cinnamon
- 1 teaspoon baking soda
- Pinch salt
- ½ cup old-fashioned oats (gluten-free)

Instructions:

1. Preheat your oven to a temperature of 375°F and line a muffin pan with paper liners.
2. Whisk together the flaxseed and water together in a bowl then let rest 5 minutes.
3. Heat the coconut oil over the medium heat setting in a small saucepan.
4. Add the apples and toss them with cinnamon then cook for 9 to 10 minutes until they are tender.
5. Remove the apples from heat and set the saucepan aside.
6. Combine the almond milk, applesauce, coconut sugar, oil, and the vanilla extract in a mixing bowl.
7. Whisk in the flax mixture until it is smooth and combined.
8. In a separate bowl, sift together the gluten-free flour blend, cinnamon, and baking soda with the salt.

9. Whisk the dry ingredients into the wet ingredients until smooth and then carefully fold in the oats and the sautéed apples.

10. Spoon the batter into the prepared muffin pan, filling the cups completely.

11. Bake for 18 to 22 minutes until a knife inserted in the center comes out clean.

12. Cool the muffins for 5 minutes in the pan then turn out onto wire racks to cool completely.

Spinach, Pepper and Mushroom Frittata
Servings: 6 to 8

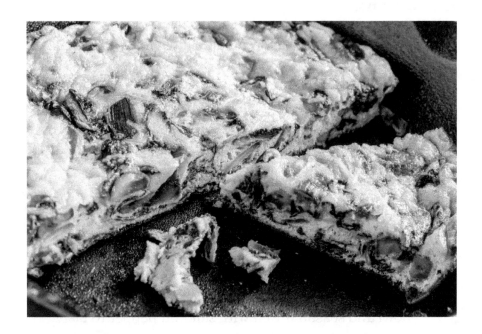

Ingredients:

- 3 teaspoons coconut oil
- 3 cups sliced baby bella mushrooms
- 1 medium red bell pepper, sliced
- 1 clove minced garlic
- Salt and pepper to taste
- 4 ounces baby spinach, chopped
- 8 large eggs, whisked well
- 2 tablespoons unsweetened almond milk

- ¼ cup fresh grated asiago cheese

Instructions:

1. Heat the coconut oil on the medium-high heat setting in a large ovenproof skillet.
2. Add the mushrooms and cook for 3 to 5 minutes until they begin to sweat.
3. Stir in the red bell pepper and garlic then season with salt and pepper to taste.
4. Cook for 1 to 2 minutes more then add in the spinach.
5. Let the spinach cook for 1 minute or so until just wilted then remove the skillet from the heat.
6. Beat together the almond milk and eggs in a mixing bowl and season it well with salt and pepper to taste.
7. Stir in the spinach, red pepper and mushroom mixture along with the cheese until well combined.
8. Reheat the skillet on the medium heat setting until very hot.
9. Pour in the egg and vegetable mixture and swirl the pan to spread the mixture evenly.
10. Cook for 4 to 5 minutes, stirring occasionally, until the eggs along the bottom of are set.
11. Reduce the temperature to low and cover the skillet then cook for about 10 minutes, shaking the pan gently every 2 minutes to distribute the ingredients.

12. Preheat the broiler in your oven then uncover the skillet and transfer it to the oven.

13. Broil for 1 to 2 minutes until the top of the frittata is set.

14. Remove the skillet to a cutting board and cool for 8 to 10 minutes before serving.

Lunch Recipes

Paleo Roasted Butternut Squash Soup
Servings: 6 to 8

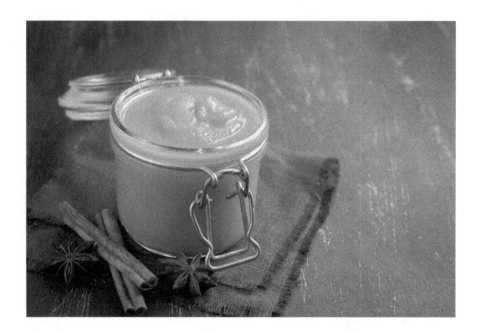

Ingredients:

- 2 medium butternut squashes
- Salt and pepper to taste
- 2 tablespoons olive oil
- 1 small sweet onion, chopped
- 1 large apple, cored and chopped

- 3 teaspoons fresh chopped sage
- 3 cups canned vegetable broth
- 2 cups water
- 6 tablespoons canned coconut milk

Instructions:

1. Preheat the oven to 425°F.
2. Cut the squash in half and carefully scoop out the seeds.
3. Place the butternut squash halves in a glass dish and then spray with cooking spray and sprinkle it well with salt and pepper.
4. Roast for 50 to 60 minutes until very tender then set it aside until cool enough to handle.
5. Scoop the squash flesh out of the skin into a bowl.
6. Heat the olive oil in a stockpot over medium heat.
7. Add the onion, apple, and sage then season with salt and pepper to taste.
8. Cook for 6 to 8 minutes until the apples and onion are tender.
9. Stir the squash into the stockpot along with the vegetable broth and water.
10. Bring the mixture to a boil and then reduce the heat - simmer on medium-low for about 15 minutes.
11. Remove the pot from heat and puree the soup using an immersion blender.

12. Whisk in the coconut milk and reheat until the soup is hot – adjust seasonings to taste.

Strawberry Balsamic Spinach Salad
Servings: 4

Ingredients:

- 6 cups fresh baby spinach, packed
- 1 to 2 cups sliced mushrooms
- ½ cup red onion, sliced thin
- 1 ½ cups diced strawberries, divided
- 2 ½ tablespoons balsamic vinegar
- 1 ½ tablespoon olive oil
- 1 teaspoon maple syrup
- Salt and pepper to taste
- Optional: Goat Cheese

Instructions:

1. Divide the spinach among four salad plates and top with sliced mushrooms and red onion.
2. Place ¼ cup diced strawberries in a food processor and sprinkle the rest over the salads.
3. Add the balsamic vinegar, olive oil, and maple syrup to the food processor.
4. Blend the mixture until smooth then season lightly with salt and pepper to taste.

5. Drizzle the salad dressing over the salads to serve.

Vegetarian Broccoli Cheddar Soup

Servings: 6 to 8

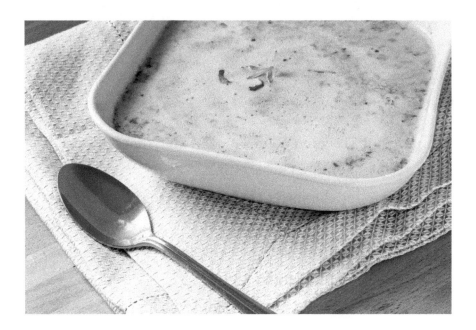

Ingredients:

- 2 tablespoons coconut oil
- ½ large white onion, coarsely chopped
- 1 teaspoon of fresh chopped thyme
- 1 teaspoon minced garlic
- ¼ cup blanched almond meal
- 2 cups of vegetable broth
- 2 ½ cups unsweetened almond milk

- ½ cup canned coconut milk (full-fat)
- 2 bay leaves
- 4 cups fresh chopped broccoli florets
- 2 cups of grated cheddar cheese
- Salt and pepper to taste

Instructions:

1. Heat the coconut oil in a medium or large saucepan on the medium-high heat setting.
2. Add in the chopped onion and cook for 6 to 8 minutes until translucent.
3. Stir in the thyme and the garlic then cook for 30 to 60 seconds until fragrant.
4. Whisk in the almond flour until smooth and cook for 1 minute.
5. Add the vegetable broth, almond milk, coconut milk, and bay leaf.
6. Bring the liquid to a boil then reduce heat slightly and simmer for about 10 minutes.
7. Stir in the broccoli and cook for 6 to 8 minutes until just tender.
8. Remove from heat then add the cheddar cheese – stir well and then sprinkle with salt and pepper to taste.
9. Let the cheese melt for a minute or two then ladle into bowls to serve.

Chicken Avocado Salad on Lettuce
Servings: 4

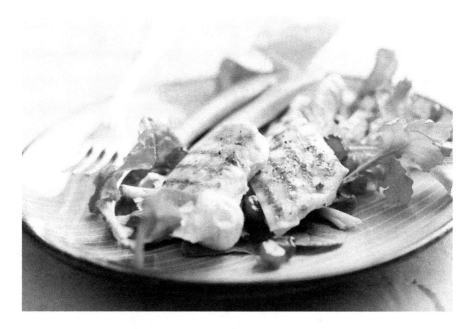

Ingredients:

- ½ cup non-fat Greek yogurt, plain
- ½ cup light mayonnaise
- 3 teaspoons fresh lemon juice
- 1 teaspoon garlic powder
- Salt and pepper to taste
- 4 cups of boneless chicken breast, cooked and shredded
- 2 ripe avocados, pitted and chopped
- 1 medium stalk celery, diced
- ¼ cup diced red onion

- 4 to 6 cups chopped romaine lettuce

Instructions:

1. Whisk together the yogurt and mayonnaise with the lemon juice and garlic in a mixing bowl.
2. Season the mixture with salt and pepper to taste.
3. Toss in the chicken, avocado, celery and red onion until coated.
4. Cover and chill the salad until cold.
5. Divide the lettuce among four salad plates.
6. Spoon the chicken avocado salad over the lettuce to serve.

Spicy Three-Bean Chili
Servings: 6 to 8

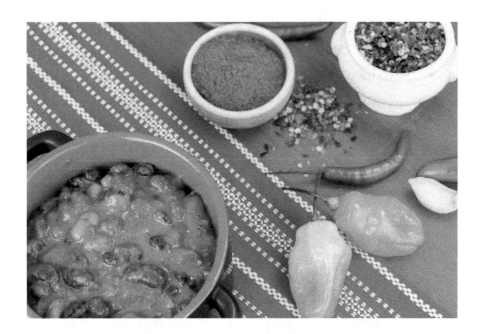

Ingredients:

- 2 tablespoons olive oil
- 3 ½ tablespoons tomato paste
- 2 ½ tablespoons chili powder
- 1 chipotle chili in adobo, drained and chopped
- ½ teaspoon cayenne pepper
- 1 ¼ cups water
- 2 (14.5-ounce cans) diced tomatoes
- 1 (15-ounce) can black beans, drained then rinsed

- 1 (15-ounce) can red kidney beans, drained then rinsed
- 1 (15-ounce) can garbanzo beans, drained then rinsed
- 1 (15-ounce) can whole-kernel corn, drained then rinsed
- 2 cups of cooked brown rice
- Diced red onion, to serve
- Shredded cheese, to serve

Instructions:

1. Heat the olive oil in a large saucepan on the medium-high heat setting.
2. Add the tomato paste, chili powder, chipotle chili and cayenne and cook for 2 or 3 minutes, stirring often.
3. Stir in the water, tomatoes, beans, and corn.
4. Bring the chili mixture to a boil and then reduce heat and simmer on medium-low for about 22 to 25 minutes.
5. Stir in the rice and cook for 5 minutes or until heated through.
6. Serve the chili hot topped with diced red onion and shredded cheddar cheese.

Spinach Salad with Hot Bacon Dressing
Servings: 4

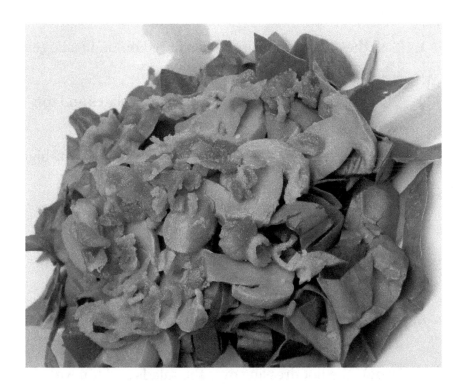

Ingredients:

- 8 ounces fresh baby spinach, chopped
- 1 cup sliced mushrooms
- ½ small red onion, sliced thin
- ½ lbs. uncooked bacon, chopped
- 3 ½ tablespoons red wine vinegar
- 1 teaspoon Dijon mustard

- Salt and pepper to taste

Instructions:

1. Toss the spinach, mushrooms and red onion in a large salad bowl.
2. Divide the spinach mixture among four plates and top with sliced egg.
3. Heat the bacon in a medium skillet on the medium-high heat setting.
4. Cook the bacon until crisp then remove the bacon to paper towels and drain.
5. Pour the bacon fat into a small saucepan and whisk in the vinegar and mustard.
6. Whisk the mixture until smooth then season lightly with salt and pepper to taste.
7. Drizzle the hot dressing over the salads and top with chopped bacon to serve.

Slow-Cooker Chicken Vegetable Stew
Servings: 6 to 8

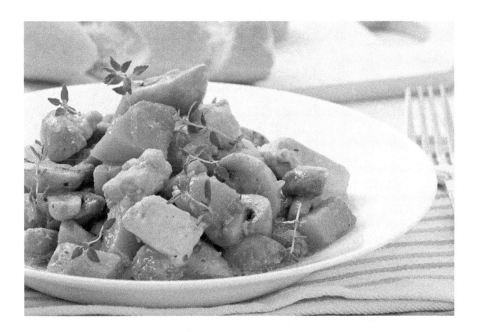

Ingredients:

- 1 ½ tablespoons coconut oil
- 1 ½ lbs. boneless chicken thighs
- Salt and pepper to taste
- 4 medium Yukon gold potatoes, diced
- 1 large sweet onion, chopped
- 2 cups of sliced white mushrooms
- 1 ½ cups chopped carrots
- 1 cup sliced celery

- 1 cup chicken or vegetable broth
- 1 ½ cups of canned tomato sauce
- 3 teaspoons fresh chopped rosemary
- ½ tablespoon minced garlic

Instructions:

1. Heat the coconut oil in a large skillet on the medium-high heat setting.
2. Season the chicken thighs with salt and pepper to taste then place them in the skillet.
3. Cook the chicken thighs for 2 to 3 minutes on both sides until they are browned.
4. Combine the potatoes with the onion, mushrooms, celery and carrots in a slow cooker.
5. Place the browned chicken on top of the vegetables.
6. Whisk together the chicken broth, tomato sauce, rosemary and garlic then pour into the slow cooker.
7. Cover the slow cooker and cook on high heat for 4 to 5 hours until the chicken thighs are cooked through and the vegetables are tender.

Vegetarian Greek-Style Chopped Salad
Servings: 4

Ingredients:

- 6 cups fresh chopped romaine lettuce
- ¼ cup fresh-squeezed lemon juice
- 2 tablespoons high-quality balsamic vinegar
- 2 ½ tablespoons olive oil
- 1 clove minced garlic
- Salt and pepper to taste
- 1 ½ cups cherry tomatoes, quartered
- 1 large seedless cucumber, diced
- 1 medium red pepper, cored and chopped
- ½ cup diced red onion
- ½ cup sliced Kalamata olives
- 1 cup crumbled up feta cheese
- Dried oregano, to serve

Instructions:

1. Divide the lettuce among four salad plates and set aside.
2. Whisk together the lemon juice with the olive oil and the vinegar and garlic in a small mixing bowl.

3. Season the dressing with salt and pepper to taste.

4. Combine the tomatoes, cucumber, bell pepper, onion, and the olives in a large bowl.

5. Toss with the salad dressing and then season the salad with salt and pepper to taste.

6. Divide the vegetable mixture among the four salad plates, spreading it evenly over the lettuce.

7. Top the salads with crumbled feta and a sprinkle of dried oregano to serve.

Dinner Recipes

Coconut-Crusted Haddock Fillets
Servings: 4

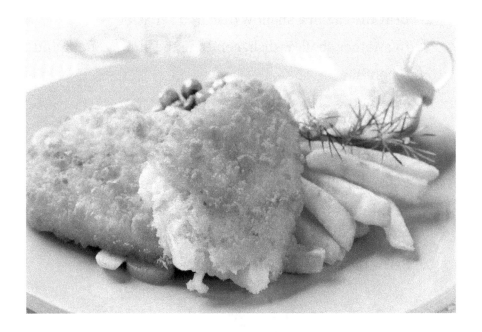

Ingredients:

- 1 large egg, beaten
- ¼ cup blanched almond flour
- ½ cup unsweetened shredded coconut
- 4 (6-ounce) boneless haddock fillets
- Salt and pepper to taste

- Lemon wedges

Instructions:

1. Preheat the oven to a temperature of 350°F and line a rimmed cookie sheet with parchment.
2. Beat the egg in a shallow dish and set aside.
3. In another shallow dish, combine the almond flour and coconut.
4. Season the fillets with salt and pepper.
5. Dip the fillets in the egg then dredge them in the coconut mixture.
6. Place the fillets on the baking sheet and bake for 15 to 18 minutes until the flesh flakes easily when you use a fork.
7. Serve the fillets hot with a lemon wedge.

Rosemary Roasted Chicken with Veggies
Servings: 6 to 8

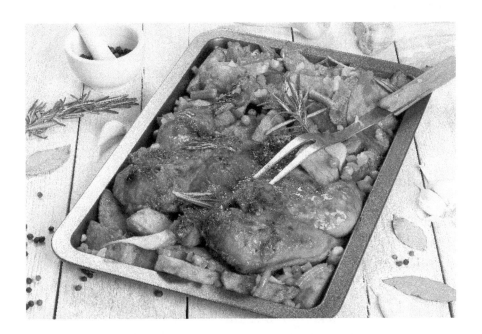

Ingredients:

- 4 tablespoons melted coconut oil, divided
- 2 medium to large sweet potatoes, chopped
- 1 large yellow onion, chopped
- 1 cup of peas
- 1 cup chopped baby carrots
- Salt and pepper to taste
- 2 ½ to 3 lbs. chicken drumsticks and thighs
- ¼ cup chicken or vegetable broth

- 2 tablespoons fresh chopped rosemary

Instructions:

1. Preheat the oven to 400°F.
2. Heat two tablespoons of oil in a medium or large skillet on the medium heat setting.
3. Add the chopped sweet potatoes, onion, broccoli and carrots – cook for 4 to 5 minutes, seasoning with salt and pepper to taste.
4. Spread the vegetables in a large rectangular glass baking dish.
5. Reheat the skillet with the remaining oil and season the chicken with salt and pepper to taste.
6. Add the chicken to the skillet and let it cook for 2 to 3 minutes on each side until browned.
7. Arrange the chicken on top of the vegetables then drizzle with chicken broth.
8. Sprinkle with rosemary and roast for 30 minutes.
9. Stir the vegetables gently and then turn the chicken then roast for another 25 to 30 minutes until the juices of the chicken run clear.

Spicy Bacon-Wrapped Scallops
Servings: 4 to 6

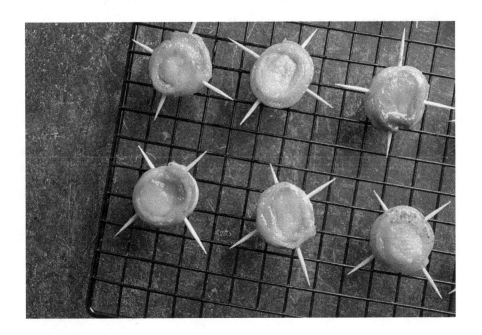

Ingredients:

- 1 lbs. uncooked sea scallops
- 1 teaspoon chili powder
- ½ teaspoon garlic powder
- ½ teaspoon paprika
- ¼ teaspoon cayenne
- Salt and pepper to taste
- ½ to 1 lbs. uncooked bacon, sliced thin

Instructions:

1. Preheat the broiler in your oven to high heat.

2. Combine the chili powder, garlic powder, paprika, and cayenne – season with salt and pepper.

3. Rinse the scallops well in cool water and then pat them dry with paper towels.

4. Wrap each skillet in a slice of bacon, securing it with a toothpick.

5. Arrange the scallops on a roasting pan and sprinkle with the seasoning mix.

6. Broil for 2 to 3 minutes on each side until the bacon is nicely crisp and the scallops cooked through.

Garlic Herb-Roasted Lamb Chops
Servings: 4 to 6

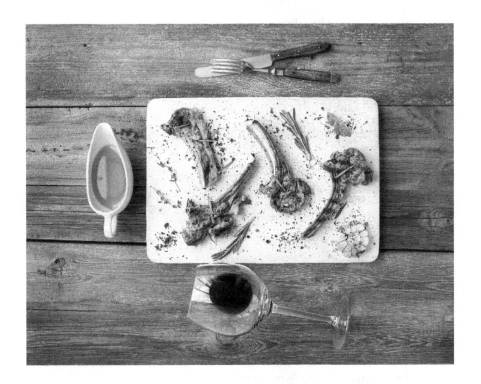

Ingredients:

- 3 cloves minced garlic
- 1 tablespoon of fresh rosemary, chopped
- 1 teaspoon fresh chopped thyme
- 2 tablespoons of olive oil, divided
- Salt and pepper to taste
- 6 bone-in lamb chops, about 1 ¼ inches thick

Instructions:

1. Preheat the oven to 400°F.

2. Place the garlic, rosemary and thyme in a bowl then mash it gently with a fork.

3. Stir in 1 tablespoon olive oil until the herb mixture is well combined.

4. Season the lamb chops with salt and pepper to taste.

5. Heat the remaining oil in an ovenproof skillet over high heat.

6. Spread the garlic herb mixture over the lamb chops then add them to the skillet.

7. Cook the lamb chops for 3 minutes on each side then move the ovenproof skillet into the oven.

8. Roast the lamb chops for 10 minutes until medium-rare.

9. Remove the lamb chops to a cutting board and let rest for 5 minutes before serving.

Vegetarian Fried Zucchini Fritters
Servings: 4 to 6

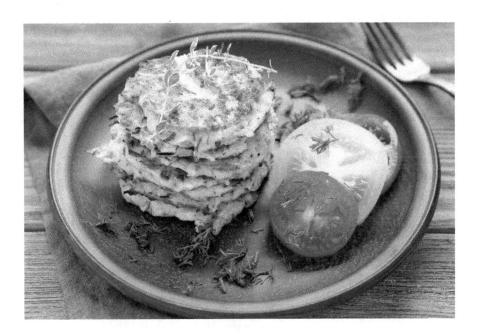

Ingredients:

- 2 medium zucchinis, ends trimmed
- Salt, as needed
- 1 cup non-fat Greek yogurt, plain
- ¼ cup sour cream
- 2 tablespoons fresh chopped dill
- 4 green onions, sliced thin
- ¼ cup fresh chopped parsley
- ¼ cup blanched almond flour

- ½ cup grated asiago cheese
- 1 large egg, beaten
- Salt and pepper to taste
- Olive oil, as needed

Instructions:

1. Grate the zucchini and spread it in a large colander.
2. Sprinkle liberally with salt then let rest for 16 to 20 minutes.
3. Whisk together the yogurt with the sour cream and the dill in a mixing bowl then set aside.
4. Press as much moisture from the grated zucchini as you can and then transfer it to a mixing bowl.
5. Stir in the green onions, parsley, almond flour, parmesan cheese and egg.
6. Season the mixture to taste with salt and pepper and stir well.
7. Heat the oil in a large skillet on the medium-high heat setting.
8. Drop the zucchini mixture into the heated oil using about ¼ cup per fritter.
9. Fry the fritters for 3 to 4 minutes until golden brown on each side.
10. Drain the fritters on paper towel.

11. Serve the fritters warm with a spoonful of the yogurt-dill mixture.

Baked Swordfish with Mango Salsa
Servings: 4

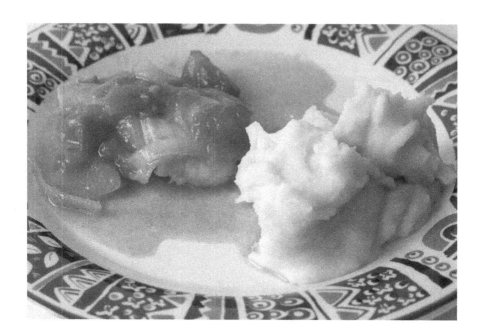

Ingredients:

- 4 (6-ounce) boneless swordfish steaks
- Olive oil, as needed
- Salt and pepper to taste
- 1 ripe mango, pitted and diced
- ½ cup chopped pineapple
- ½ small red pepper, cored and chopped
- ¼ cup diced red onion
- 2 tablespoons freshly squeezed lime juice

- 2 tablespoons chopped cilantro
- 2 Potatoes

Instructions:

1. Preheat the oven to 350°F.
2. Brush the swordfish with olive oil and season with salt and pepper to taste.
3. Place the fillets on a parchment-lined baking sheet and bake for 15 to 18 minutes until the flesh flakes easily with a fork.
4. Meanwhile, combine the mango, pineapple, red pepper and onion in a medium bowl.
5. Toss in the lime juice, cilantro, salt and pepper.
6. Serve the swordfish steaks hot topped with the mango salsa.
7. Serve with smashed potatoes

Vegan Portobello Burger
Servings: 4

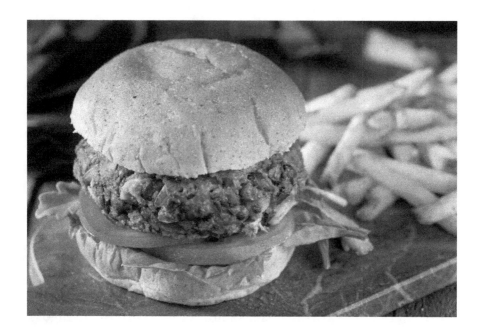

Ingredients:

- 4 large Portobello mushroom caps
- Olive oil, as needed
- Salt and pepper to taste
- 4 vegan sandwich buns, toasted
- 4 tablespoons fresh basil pesto
- 1 ½ cups fresh arugula

Instructions:

1. Preheat the grill to the medium-high heat setting and brush the grates with olive oil.
2. Remove the stems from the mushroom caps and brush both sides with olive oil.
3. Season the mushroom caps with salt and pepper to taste then place them on the preheated grill gill-side down.
4. Grill for 4 minutes and then turn the mushroom caps over.
5. Cover the grill and cook for another 3 to 4 minutes until tender.
6. Spread about 1 tablespoon pesto on the top half of each sandwich bun.
7. Place one grilled mushroom cap onto the bottom half of each sandwich bun.
8. Top the mushrooms with fresh arugula and the top half of the buns. Serve hot.

Paleo Homestyle Meatloaf
Servings: 4 to 6

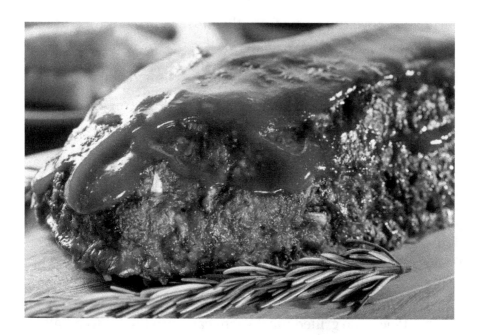

Ingredients:

- 1 tablespoon coconut oil
- 3 to 4 cloves minced garlic
- 2 cups white mushrooms, diced
- 1 cup yellow onion, chopped
- Salt and pepper to taste
- 2 lbs. lean ground beef
- 1 large egg, beaten
- 1 teaspoon dried oregano

- 1 teaspoon dried thyme
- ½ cup paleo-friendly ketchup
- 2 teaspoons maple syrup

Instructions:

1. Preheat the oven to 350°F.
2. Heat the coconut oil in a large skillet on the medium-high heat setting.
3. Stir in the garlic along with the mushrooms and onion.
4. Cook for 6 to 8 minutes until the onion is nearly translucent and then transfer to a mixing bowl.
5. Stir in the ground beef, egg, oregano, thyme, salt and pepper.
6. Spread the meat and vegetable mixture in a greased loaf pan, pressing it down evenly.
7. Whisk together the ketchup and the maple syrup then spread it over the meatloaf.
8. Bake for about an hour until the internal temperature of the meatloaf reaches 155°F.
9. Cool the meatloaf for 10 minutes then slice to serve.

Snacks and Desserts

Baked Cinnamon Apple Chips
Servings: 4 to 6

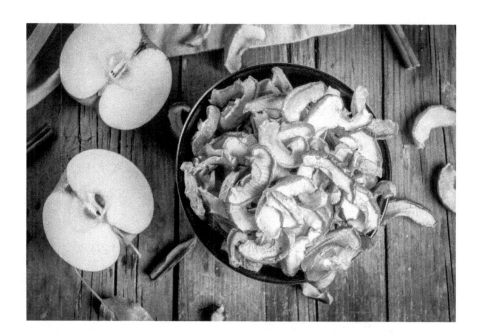

Ingredients:

- 3 to 4 large ripe apples
- Ground cinnamon, to taste

Instructions:

1. Preheat the oven to 220°F and line two rimmed baking sheets with parchment paper.
2. Slice the apples as thinly as possible using a mandolin and discard the seeds.
3. Spread the apple slices on the baking sheets in a single layer.
4. Sprinkle liberally with cinnamon.
5. Bake for 1 hour then carefully flip the apple slices and bake for another hour.
6. Turn off the oven and let the apple slices cool until crisp.

Fudgy Coconut Flour Brownies

Servings: 12 to 14

Ingredients:

- 1 cup unsweetened almond milk
- ¼ cup flaxseed meal
- 1 cup chopped dark chocolate
- ½ cup honey
- 3 tablespoons coconut sugar
- 3 tablespoons of coconut oil

- ½ tablespoon pure vanilla extract
- 2/3 cup coconut flour
- 2 ½ tablespoons arrowroot powder
- 1 teaspoon baking powder
- ¼ teaspoon of baking soda
- Pinch salt

Instructions:

1. Preheat the oven to 365°F and line the bottom of an 8-by-8-inch glass baking dish with parchment.
2. Place the almond milk in a saucepan and heat until warm then remove from heat.
3. Whisk in the flaxseed and chocolate, stirring until the dark chocolate is completely melted.
4. Add the honey, sugar, coconut oil and vanilla extract then whisk smooth.
5. Set the mixture aside for 5 minutes.
6. In a medium mixing bowl, stir together the coconut flour and arrowroot powder with the baking powder, the baking soda and the salt.
7. Whisk the dry ingredients into the wet in small batches, stirring smooth after each addition.
8. Spread the blended brownie batter evenly in the prepared glass dish.

9. Bake for 24 to 26 minutes until the center is set then cool completely before cutting into squares to serve.

Creamy Spinach Artichoke Dip
Servings: 12 to 14

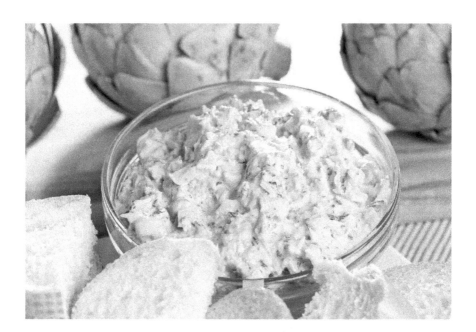

Ingredients:

- 1 (10-ounce) bag frozen spinach, thawed and squeezed dry
- 1 (14-ounce) can artichoke hearts, drained then chopped
- 1 cup grated parmesan cheese
- 1 cup fresh grated asiago cheese
- 1 (8-ounce) package of cream cheese, room temperature
- 2/3 cup regular sour cream

- 1/3 cup light mayonnaise
- 1 tablespoon minced garlic

Instructions:

1. Preheat the oven to a temperature of 375°F.
2. Stir together the spinach, artichoke hearts, parmesan and asiago cheese in a mixing bowl.
3. In a separate bowl, whisk together the cream cheese along with the sour cream, mayonnaise and garlic.
4. Stir the spinach mixture into the cream cheese mixture until well combined.
5. Spread the mixture in a round casserole dish and bake the mixture for 25 to 30 minutes until hot.

Avocado Chocolate Mousse
Servings: 6 to 8

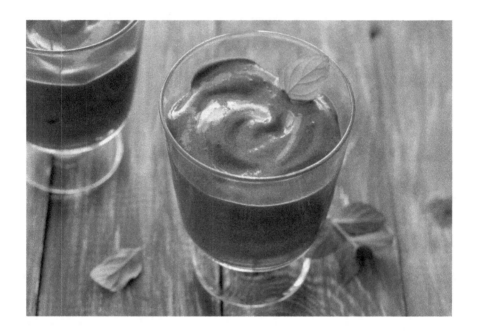

Ingredients:

- ¾ cups dark chocolate chips
- 5 large ripe avocados, pitted and chopped
- ¾ cup unsweetened cocoa powder
- ¾ cup raw honey
- ½ cup unsweetened almond milk
- 1 tablespoon pure vanilla extract
- Pinch salt

Instructions:

1. Place the chocolate chips in a double boiler on the medium-low heat setting.
2. Stir the mixture until the chocolate is melted then set aside.
3. Combine the avocado, cocoa powder, honey, almond milk and the vanilla in a regular food processor.
4. Add the melted dark chocolate along with a pinch of salt.
5. Blend the mixture until smooth and well combined.
6. Spoon into dessert cups and chill for 4 to 6 hours before serving.

Vegan Paleo Baked Sweet Potato Wedges
Servings: 4 to 6

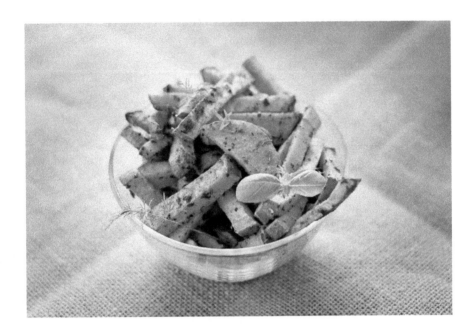

Ingredients:

- 6 medium to large sweet potatoes, peeled
- 2 tablespoons olive oil
- 1 teaspoon smoked paprika
- Salt and pepper to taste

Instructions:

1. Preheat the oven to a temperature of 450°F and line two rimmed baking sheets with parchment.
2. Cut the sweet potatoes into wedges about ¼-inch thick.
3. Toss the sweet potatoes with the olive oil, paprika, salt and pepper.
4. Spread the sweet potatoes in a single layer on top of the rimmed baking sheets.
5. Bake for 20 minutes, turning the sweet potatoes halfway through, until the edges are browned.
6. Cool for 10 minutes before you serve the wedges.

Flourless Chocolate Cake

Servings: 8

Ingredients:

- 6 ounces chopped dark chocolate
- ¾ cup coconut oil
- 1 cup plus 3 tablespoons granulated sugar
- 4 large eggs, whisked well
- ¾ cup unsweetened cocoa powder

Instructions:

1. Preheat the oven to 375°F and grease 8 cups in a regular muffin pan with cooking spray.
2. Melt the chocolate and coconut oil in a double boiler on the medium-low heat setting.
3. Stir the mixture smooth and remove from heat.
4. Whisk in the sugar then whisk in the eggs, one egg at a time.
5. Sprinkle the cocoa powder over the mixture and whisk it in until just combined.
6. Divide the mixture among the muffin pan cups.
7. Bake for 18 to 22 minutes until a crust forms on the top of the cakes.

8. Cool the cakes for 5 minutes in the pan then turn out onto a wire rack and serve warm.

Roasted Red Pepper Hummus
Servings: 10 to 12

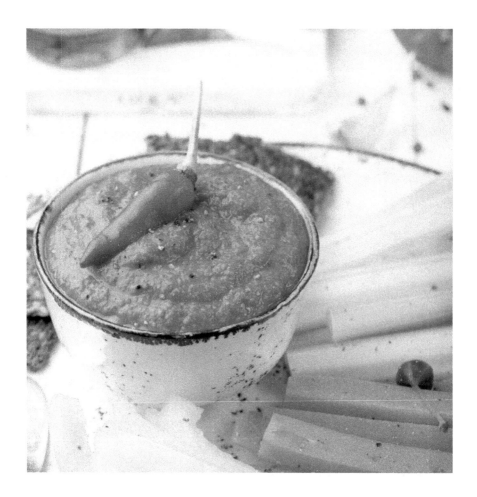

Ingredients:

- 1 (15.5-ounce) can chickpeas, rinsed and drained
- 1 (6-ounce) jar of roasted red peppers, chopped

- 3 cloves minced garlic
- ½ jalapeno, seeded and minced
- Salt and pepper to taste
- 4 tablespoons olive oil
- Water, as needed

Instructions:

1. Combine the chickpeas, roasted red pepper, garlic and jalapeno in a food processor.
2. Blend the mixture until smooth then season with salt and pepper to taste.
3. With the food processor running, drizzle in the oil.
4. Blend until the hummus reaches the desired consistency, thinning with water if needed.
5. Serve the hummus with sliced veggies for dipping.

Vegan Oatmeal Raisin Cookies
Servings: 28 to 32

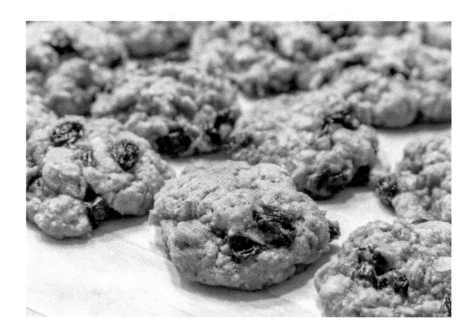

Ingredients:

- 3 ½ cups toasted walnut halves
- 1 ½ cups gluten-free flour blend
- 1 cup coconut sugar
- 2 teaspoons of baking soda
- 1 ½ teaspoons ground cinnamon
- 4 cups gluten-free oats, divided
- 1 cup raw honey
- 6 tablespoons coconut oil, melted

- ¼ cup unsweetened almond milk
- 1 tablespoon pure vanilla extract
- 1 to 1 ½ cups seedless raisins

Instructions:

1. Preheat the oven to 350°F and line two baking sheets with sheets of parchment paper.
2. Place the walnuts in a food processor and then pulse the mixture until it forms a fine flour.
3. Combine the flour, coconut sugar, baking soda, cinnamon and 2 cups oats in a mixing bowl.
4. Add the dry ingredients to the food processor then pulse several times to combine.
5. Whisk together the honey and coconut oil with the almond milk and vanilla extract in a small mixing bowl.
6. Add the wet ingredients to the food processor and then pulse it several times until well combined.
7. Transfer the cookie dough into a large mixing bowl and then stir in the remaining gluten-free oats along with the raisins.
8. Pinch off pieces of dough (about 2 tablespoons each) and roll them into balls by hand.
9. Place the balls on the baking sheets, spacing them about 2 inches apart, and flatten gently by hand.

10. Bake for 10 minutes then cool on the baking sheet for 2 minutes.

11. Remove the cookies to a cooling rack and cool for 15 minutes before serving.

Conclusion

After reading this book it is my hope that you have a deeper understanding of what the gluten-free diet is and what benefits it can provide. While the gluten-free diet is a medical treatment for individuals with celiac disease or gluten intolerance, it can be beneficial for nearly everyone. Before you decide whether the gluten-free diet is the right choice for you, take the time to learn as much as you can about the diet including its benefits, its risks, and which foods you can and cannot eat. If you decide that the gluten-free diet is the diet for you, I hope you will try some of the recipes in this book as you transition into the diet.

Please let me know your favorites- the review section of this book is an excellent place to share your experience with other readers.

To post an honest review, please visit:

http://bit.ly/gluten-free-beginners

DON'T FORGET YOUR FREE EBOOK

Irresistible Gluten Free Desserts, Snacks & Treats

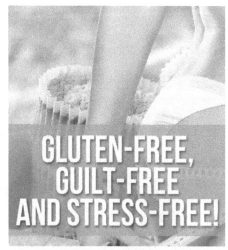

Download Link:

RELATED READING

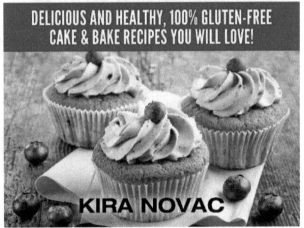

Amazon Book Page Link:

http://bit.ly/gf-baking

RELATED READING

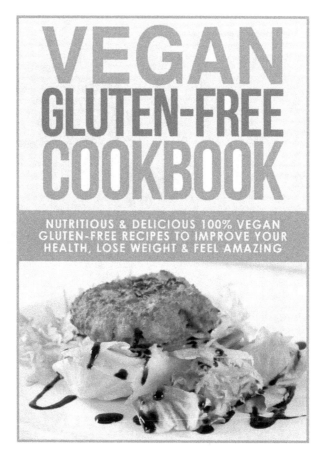

Amazon Book Page Link:

bit.ly/vegan-gluten-free

FOR MORE HEALTH BOOKS (KINDLE & PAPERBACK) BY KIRA NOVAC, PLEASE VISIT:

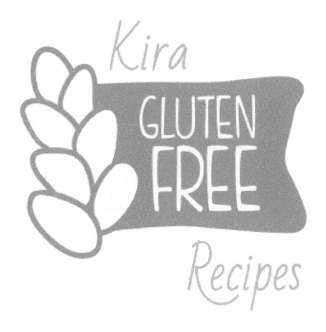

www.kiraglutenfreerecipes.com/books

Thank you for taking an interest in my work!

Kira Novac